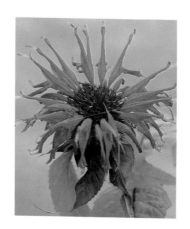

herbal teas

for health and healing

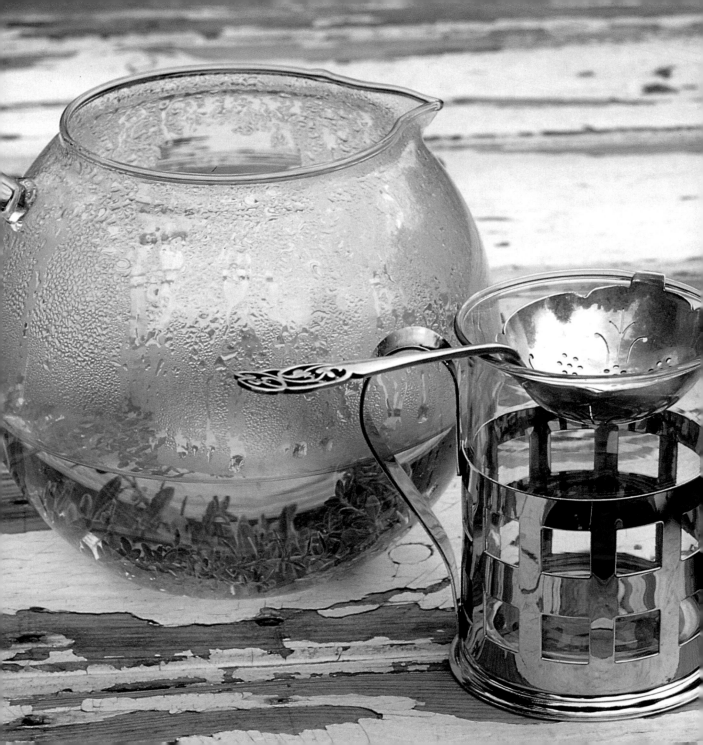

herbal teas
for health and healing

make your own natural drinks to improve zest and vitality, and to help relieve common ailments, with 50 herb and fruit infusions and 100 beautiful photographs

jessica houdret

LORENZ BOOKS

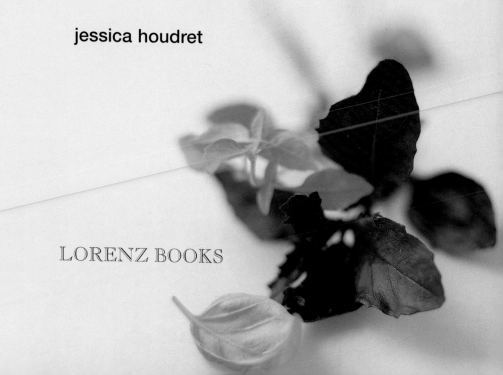

This edition is published by Lorenz Books, an imprint of Anness Publishing Ltd,
Hermes House, 88–89 Blackfriars Road, London SE1 8HA;
tel. 020 7401 2077; fax 020 7633 9499

www.lorenzbooks.com; www.annesspublishing.com

If you like the images in this book and would like to investigate using them
for publishing, promotions or advertising, please visit our website
www.practicalpictures.com for more information.

UK agent: The Manning Partnership Ltd; tel. 01225 478444;
fax 01225 478440; sales@manning-partnership.co.uk
UK distributor: Grantham Book Services Ltd;
tel. 01476 541080; fax 01476 541061; orders@gbs.tbs-ltd.co.uk
North American agent/distributor: National Book Network;
tel. 301 459 3366; fax 301 429 5746; www.nbnbooks.com
Australian agent/distributor: Pan Macmillan Australia;
tel. 1300 135 113; fax 1300 135 103; customer.service@macmillan.com.au
New Zealand agent/distributor: David Bateman Ltd;
tel. (09) 415 7664; fax (09) 415 8892

Publisher **Joanna Lorenz**
Managing Editor **Helen Sudell**
Project Editor **Simona Hill**
Copy Editor **Beverley Jollands**
Designer **Mark Latter**
Editorial Reader **Diane Ashmore**
Production Controller **Pirong Wang**

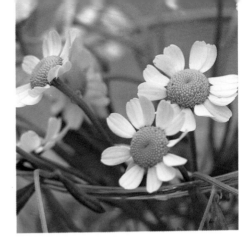

ETHICAL TRADING POLICY
Because of our ongoing ecological investment programme, you, as our customer, can
have the pleasure and reassurance of knowing that a tree is being cultivated on your
behalf to naturally replace the materials used to make the book you are holding.
For further information about this scheme, go to www.annesspublishing.com/trees

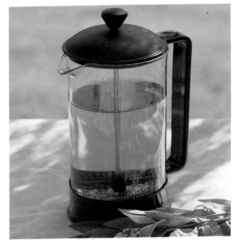

A CIP catalogue record for this book is available from the British Library.

Previously published as *Herbal Tea Remedies*

Acknowledgements
The publishers would like to thank the following photographers: Michelle Garrett, Amanda Heywood,
Don Last, Lucy Mason, Debbie Patterson and Polly Wreford. Thanks to the following contributors:
Kathy Brown, Stephanie Donaldson, Mark Evans, Tessa Evelegh, Nicola Graimes, Sue Hawkey,
Jessica Houdret, Andrea Jones, Gilly Love, Liz McCauley and Peter McHoy.

Caution
The reader should not regard the recommendations, ideas and techniques described
in this book as substitutes for the advice of a qualified medical practitioner or other qualified
professional. Any use to which the recommendations, ideas and techniques are put is at the reader's
sole discretion and use.

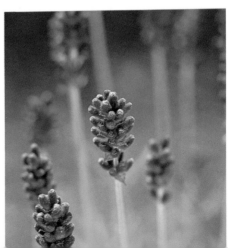

Contents

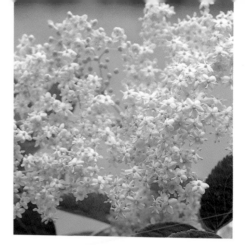

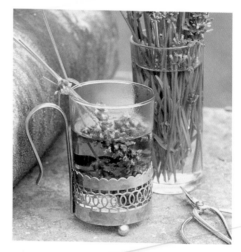

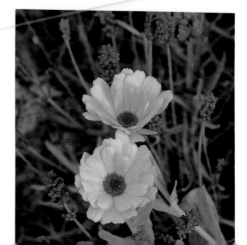

introduction

Throughout time, people have used plants not only as food but also for medicinal purposes. Traditional knowledge of herbal remedies used to be passed down the generations, but these days most of us have lost touch with the folklore of herbalism. In modern industrialized societies we consume less natural plant material than our ancestors and have a lifestyle which is a far cry from theirs. Fortunately, the herbs that our ancestors would have recognized have survived in abundance, many of which can be grown in your own garden, or even in pots or windowboxes.

Getting to know the plants growing around you can be a relaxing pleasure in itself. If you learn about the various properties of these beneficial plants, and grow those that are suited to you, you can use them to help you feel more healthy and better able to cope with everyday problems.

Herbs in history

Wall paintings dating from around 3000BC show that ancient Egyptian medicine employed herbs that remain familiar today, including juniper, mint and marjoram. The Egyptians also used herbs to flavour food, and added them to cosmetics and enbalming ointments. These skills were adopted by

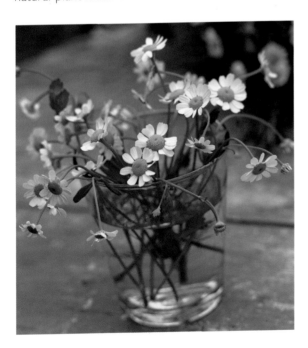

left **Chamomile, with its sedative and soothing characteristics, is one of the most beneficial herbs to have to hand.**

the Greeks and Romans, and the spread of the Roman empire meant that herbs native to the Mediterranean region were widely distributed.

After the fall of Rome, herbal knowledge in Europe was nurtured and kept alive in Christian monasteries. By the 10th century, Arab scholars learnt to distil the essential oils of plants. Their knowledge, and the plants themselves, were taken to Europe by returning Crusaders.

In Europe, the Renaissance brought advances in the study of the healing properties of plants. The 16th and 17th centuries were the age of the great herbalists, including Brunfels, Fuchs, Dodoens, Gerard and Culpeper. Huge quantities of plants, many of which were used by the Native Americans, arrived in Europe from America. Meanwhile, other herbs, including parsley, savory and thyme, were taken to America by early settlers keen to plant familiar gardens. Herbs were also widely used in cookery and perfumery, but the line drawn between pleasure and health was a narrow one – it was generally accepted that a fragrant smell was in itself proof against infection.

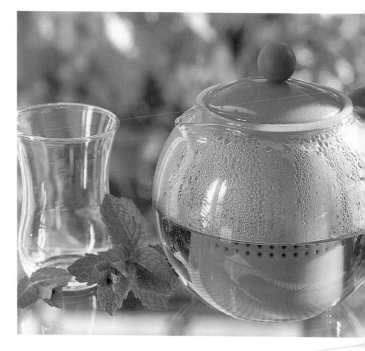

above **Peppermint tea aids digestion, and soothes a cold, with its decongestant, antiseptic qualities.**

Until the 18th century, botany and medicine were closely allied, but with the rise of modern scientific enquiry they became separate disciplines and synthetic drugs began their ascendancy. In the 21st century, there is an increasing recognition by scientists of the value of plants as the basis for drugs to combat major diseases. However, where

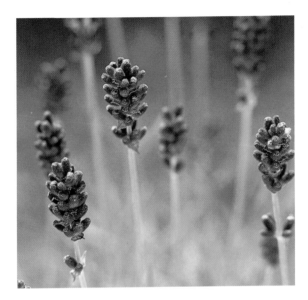

above Lavender is instantly recognizable by its perfume, and is one of the most widely used herbs.

herbalists use the whole plant for treatment, the drugs under development by pharmaceutical companies depend on isolating and copying active plant constituents as a basis for their treatments.

Herbs in the diet

The connection with diet and health is undisputed, and herbs play a key role. Many of them have a direct medicinal action that you can take into account when cooking with them. Garlic, for example, is thought to ward off colds and flu, lower cholesterol and reduce the risk of heart disease. Thyme, which is high in antioxidants, has been linked to slowing the ageing process, and also has antiseptic properties. Pungent ginger counteracts nausea and aids the absorption of other foods.

It is well documented that the consumption of certain foods boosts the immune system. The key is to eat plenty of fresh fruit, vegetables, whole grains and vegetable oils. All contain antioxidants which counteract the unstable and potentially harmful free radicals formed by the body's metabolism through stress, pollution and ageing.

Why herbs are good for you

Herbs have a valuable contribution to make, since many contain vital antioxidants, vitamins, minerals and trace elements. Don't just think of them as flavourings: you can make herbs such as parsley, watercress, nettles and mint the main ingredients of delicious soups and salads. Herbs, like people, are complex and variable organic structures made up of many parts. Each plant contains many different constituents, which combine to give it a unique taste and range of actions. Particularly active constituents have been isolated and copied by pharmacists to produce medicines such as aspirin. However, using the whole plant has a more subtle effect and generates fewer side effects.

Drinking herbal teas

Very simple remedies can easily be made using fresh or dried herbs, and substituting herbal teas for stimulating drinks such as tea, coffee and cola will help you to relax and reduce tension.

Herbal teas are also called infusions or tisanes, and are a simple and effective way of extracting the goodness and flavour from the aerial parts of herbs – the leaves, soft stems and flowers. You can use either fresh or dried herbs to make a tea (use twice as much fresh plant material as dried). If you find the taste of some herb teas a problem, they can be sweetened with a little honey or flavoured by stirring them with a licorice root stick; you can also try adding slices of lemon or fresh ginger.

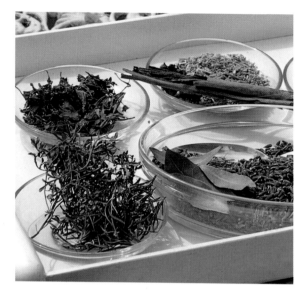

above **Your knowledge of herbal remedies will increase if you grow, harvest and dry your own herbs.**

CAUTIONS

- Avoid all strong herbal teas during the first three months of pregnancy.
- Do not give peppermint or sage tea to children under four years of age.
- Do not take licorice if you suffer from high blood pressure.
- Do not take vervain if you have liver disease.
- Do not exceed recommended quantities for ingredients and frequency of drinking.

growing herbs

The most satisfying way to obtain fresh herbs is to grow them yourself. If you have a garden, aromatic herbs can be included in your general planting scheme, in an ornamental border, or in a vegetable plot. However, a designated herb garden always makes a rewarding feature. Most herbs are not fussy or difficult to grow, but will prefer a location in full sun.

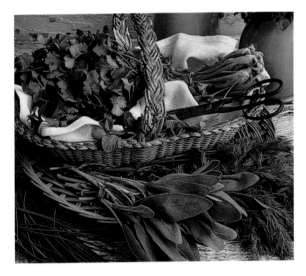

above **Use herbs as soon as they are picked so that the essential oils do not evaporate.**

Growing herbs in containers has many advantages, particularly where space is limited. Growing a single species in a container gives plants room to develop and to provide plenty of leafy growth. For larger specimens, such as sage, rosemary and lemon verbena, it is essential that they do not have to share a pot if they are to be left undisturbed for several years.

Good drainage is one of the keys to success. Containers should have a generous layer of broken pots in the base and should be filled with an open planting mix containing plenty of sand or gravel. If you are planting your herbs in open ground, lighten heavy clay soil by digging in some sand or gravel.

Some herbs adapt well to being grown indoors, and this is one way of cultivating tender herbs successfully. Give indoor plants as much natural light as possible and regular liquid feeds in summer, but do not overwater them. A supply of herbs on the kitchen windowsill is very convenient, but you should alternate pots with others standing outside.

harvesting herbs

Home-grown herbs can be harvested continuously. Once established, most herbs will grow strongly enough to allow plenty of repeat picking, which encourages new growth in healthy, well-cared-for plants. The best time to harvest depends on the herb and the part of it that you require – leaf, flower or seed. A few evergreen herbs, such as rosemary and sage, may be lightly picked when dormant.

Choose a fine, sunny day, preferably before noon, for picking herbs, so that the essential oil content, which gives the plant its flavour and scent, is at its best. Use sharp scissors so as not to damage the plants, and pick only prime material from plants that are at their peak. Pick herbs as you need them.

• Leaves should be picked before the plants come into flower, when their flavour and texture are at their peak. Pick small-leaved herbs stem by stem and strip them later. Larger leaves can be picked individually.

• Flowers should be cut soon after they have opened, when they are at their best. Pick single blooms or flower-heads as appropriate and strip off the petals or florets when you spread them out to dry. Lavender should be picked with a long stem.

• Seeds must be picked as soon as they are ripe, when they are no longer green, but before they fall. This means watching them carefully, as they can ripen and disperse very quickly.

below **Pick herbs in quantities you can deal with at one time – don't leave them in heaps waiting to be processed, as they deteriorate quickly.**

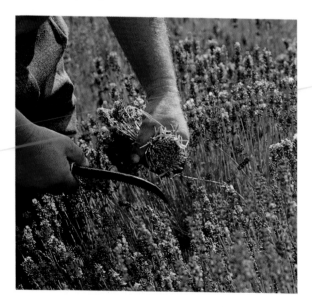

drying and storing herbs

Herbs are bountiful, putting on rapid growth during the summer, so there is plenty to harvest. When drying herbs, the aim is to remove the moisture without sacrificing the volatile oil content. Drying has to be rapid so that the plants do not decay, but not so fast that the oils are destroyed by heat.

below **Dry herbs in bunches in a warm, dry place, away from direct sunlight.**

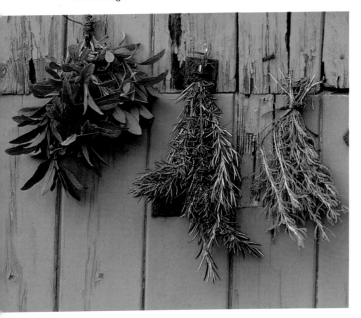

You need to achieve the right temperature and low humidity. An airing cupboard is ideal, and a clean, dry shed can also work well: both can be kept dark to preserve the colour of the herbs. Avoid washing herbs when you prepare them for drying – instead, brush the leaves with a pastry brush or wipe with a dry cloth – that way none of the oils are lost.

Drying green leaves

Small leaves can be dried on the stems and larger leaves individually. Spread them on slatted trays or on fine netting stretched over a frame so that air can circulate around them. Leave them in a warm dark place with some ventilation. Alternatively, tie the herbs in bunches and hang them upside down in a warm, dark, airy place. Choose a space where you can leave the herbs undisturbed for a while.

The leaves should be dry and crisp within a week. Strip the leaves from the stems, or crumble the larger ones into small pieces ready to store.

Drying flowers

Twist off the heads of large flowers and spread out the petals on paper-lined, slatted trays. Small flowers are best hung in bunches, tied with string. Enclose the heads in paper bags to exclude dust and catch any florets that fall as they dry. Put in a warm, dry, airy place and leave until papery dry.

Drying seeds

Pick seed heads with stems attached. Tie them in bunches, insert the heads in paper bags and hang them up in a warm, airy place. When they are completely dry, clean off the pods or husks and store in clearly marked envelopes or paper bags.

Storing herbs and flowers

Dried herbs and flowers deteriorate quickly, losing their aroma and colour, if they are left exposed to light and air. Store them in airtight jars and keep them in a dark, dry place.

Instead of drying herbs, store them in the freezer. This is useful for herbs such as lemon balm and parsley, which lose their flavour when dried.

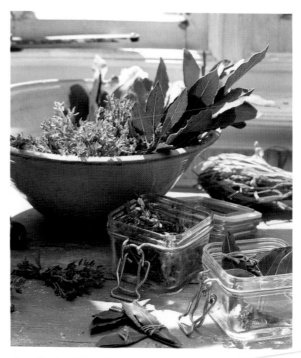

above **Herbs will keep for a long time, and will retain their colour and oils, if stored in the right conditions.**

Buying herbs

Many shops stock dried herbs, or freeze-dried herbs. This is often the best way of obtaining stocks of those herbs that are difficult to identify or hard to grow, such as hibiscus, damiana and skullcap.

making herbal teas

One of the easiest ways to benefit from the properties of a herb is to drink it as a tea. The taste of teas made from fresh or home-dried garden herbs is second to none, and you can be sure that you are getting the maximum benefit from the properties of the herbs. For most medicinal purposes, drink a cupful of the appropriate tea three times a day. Teas can be stored for up to 24 hours in the refrigerator.

Allow 30ml/2 tbsp fresh or 15ml/1 tbsp dried herbs to each 600ml/1 pint/2½ cups water. Sweeten with licorice root or honey, but never add milk.

Using a cafetière

A cafetière (press pot) is a convenient alternative to a teapot, as it cuts out the need to strain the tea. If you are using fresh herbs, wash them first.

1 Put fresh or dried herbs, in the quantities given, into a warmed cafetière and pour on boiling water.

2 Replace the lid and leave to brew for the recommended time.

3 Push down the plunger when the infusion is strong enough to serve.

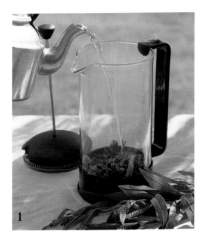

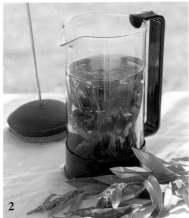

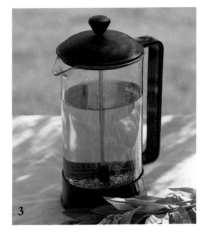

Making a decoction

Infusing in boiling water is not enough to extract the constituents from roots or bark, such as valerian or licorice. Harder plant material needs to be boiled and the resulting liquid is called a decoction. Use a pan that is not aluminium to prepare decoctions.

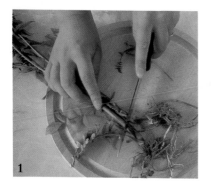
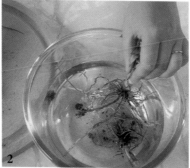
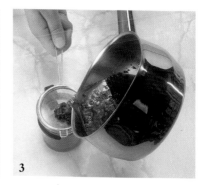

1 Roots and barks need to be harvested in the autumn and prepared for use. Trim the aerial parts of the plant from the root and discard.

2 Wash the roots or bark thoroughly in clean water and chop into small pieces. Fill a pan with cold water and add 5ml/1 tsp of the chopped herb per cup of water. Bring to the boil and simmer for 10–15 minutes.

3 Strain off the liquid and allow to cool before drinking. It can be kept in the refrigerator for 24 hours and drunk hot or cold.

USING A TISANIÈRE

A tisanière is a cup with an integral strainer and a lid. Covering the cup with the lid prevents the properties of the herb from evaporating before you drink it. Put a sprig of fresh herb, or 5ml/ 1 tsp dried herb, into the strainer compartment and pour in boiling water. Put on the lid and leave to brew for the recommended time. Lift out the strainer before drinking the tea.

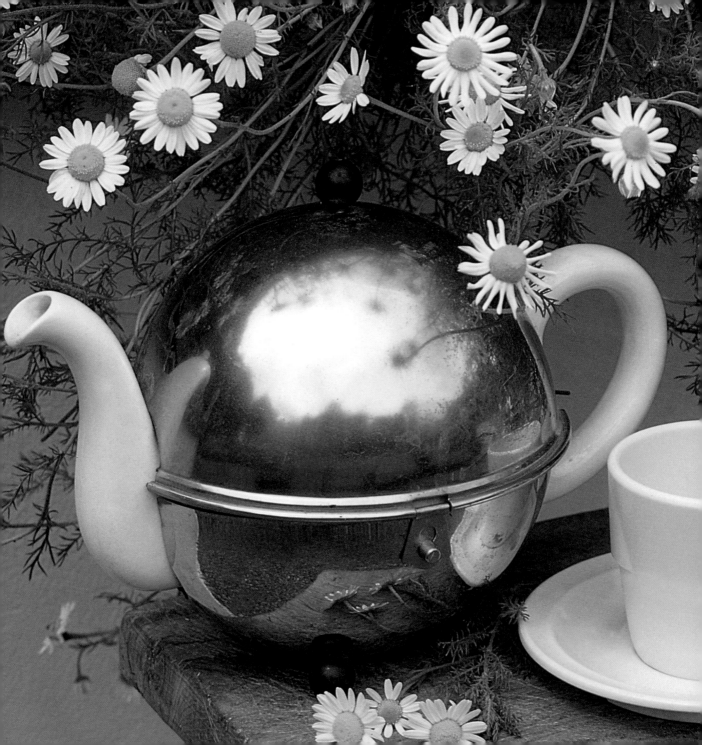

teas for digestion

Many people suffer from digestive upsets when they are subjected to anxiety. This is because external stresses stimulate the body's sympathetic nervous system to initiate its "fight or flight" response, making the heart and lungs more active and suppressing processes such as digestion and elimination. The result may be indigestion, loss of appetite, flatulence, diarrhoea or an irritable bowel. Herbal remedies can relax the nervous system and reduce spasm in the gut. Drink one cupful after a meal, but no more than two or three cups a day.

Chamomile tea

Tea made with chamomile flowers has an anti-inflammatory action and is soothing and sedative. As well as indigestion, chamomile tea can help with nausea and promote sound sleep.

The tisane can be bitter if you use too many flowers or infuse them for too long. Try making it with three or four flower-heads and add a little honey if you wish.

Recipe

30ml/2 tbsp fresh or 15ml/1 tbsp dried chamomile
600ml/1 pint/2½ cups boiling water

1 Put the chamomile into a pot and pour on the boiling water.
2 Leave to steep for four minutes, then strain.

Variation

Substitute half the chamomile with dried peppermint.

Peppermint tisane

This variety of the mint family is particularly rich in menthol, which gives it its characteristic cooling, slightly numbing taste. Just one sprig is enough to flavour a delicious tisane which has lots of peppermint flavour. Add to 250ml/8fl oz/ 1 cup of water. Drunk hot or cold, it makes a safe and palatable cure for indigestion and nausea. Combine fresh peppermint and lemon balm in equal quantities to make a pleasantly flavoured digestive tea to drink after a meal.

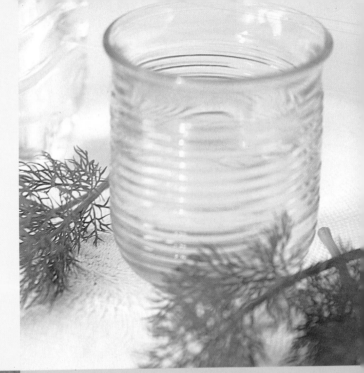

Dill tea

This ancient herb may get its common name from the Saxon word dile, to lull, because it has been used since ancient times to soothe colic in babies. It is an ingredient of "gripe water". It acts gently to ease indigestion and to regularize the system. It can safely be given to babies and young children. Allow 5ml/1 tsp lightly crushed dill seed to a 250ml/8fl oz/ 1 cup of water and boil for 10 minutes. Strain and allow to cool before drinking.

Fennel seed tea

Fennel has a mild aniseed flavour. It is a diuretic and has a calming effect on the stomach. To ease flatulence and indigestion, allow 5ml/1 tsp lightly crushed fennel seed to 250ml/8fl oz/1 cup of water and boil for 10 minutes. Strain and allow to cool before drinking. Add a slice of orange or a sliver of orange rind for extra flavour. Caraway seeds can be prepared in the same way, or combined with fennel in equal quantities.

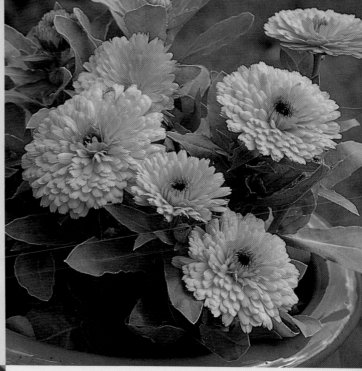

Marigold and verbena tisane

This attractive and distinctive gold and green tisane is reputed to be excellent for purifying the blood and aiding digestion. The verbena gives the tea an intensely lemony flavour and the marigold adds a peppery note. Mix 50g/2oz dried marigold petals with 25g/1oz dried lemon verbena leaves and store in an airtight container. Prepare an infusion using this mixture in the normal way, using 5ml/1 tsp to 250ml/8fl oz/1 cup of boiling water.

teas for coughs and colds

Hot, comforting herbal teas can help both to ward off winter coughs and colds and to alleviate the symptoms if you do pick up an infection. High doses of vitamin C are useful for preventing the development of colds, while the antiseptic properties of herbs such as thyme and sage can guard against the onset of secondary bacterial infections. When you are feeling shivery, you can make herbal teas extra comforting with warming additions such as slices of fresh ginger or a pinch of cayenne, both of which also have antiseptic properties. Drink one or two cups a day.

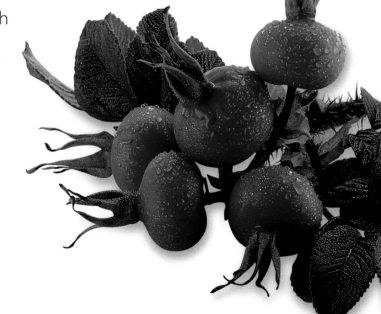

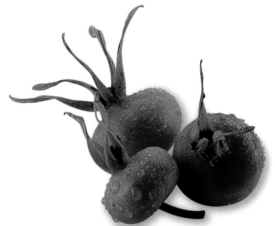

Rose-hip tea

Weight for weight rose-hips contain eight times as much vitamin C as oranges. When they are very ripe, rose-hips can be eaten raw, but a more pleasant way to enjoy them is in a sweet, astringent tea. As it is caffeine-free, rose-hip tea can be enjoyed at any time of day, either hot or chilled with an optional squeeze of lemon.

Recipe
2 tbsp crushed rose-hips
600ml / 1 pint / 2½ cups water
honey (optional)

1 Place the rose-hips in a bowl, add cold water just to cover, and leave to soak for 24 hours out of direct sunlight.

2 Bring the water to boil in a non-aluminium pan and add the rose-hips. Simmer for about 30 minutes, then strain. Add a little honey to sweeten the tea if you wish.

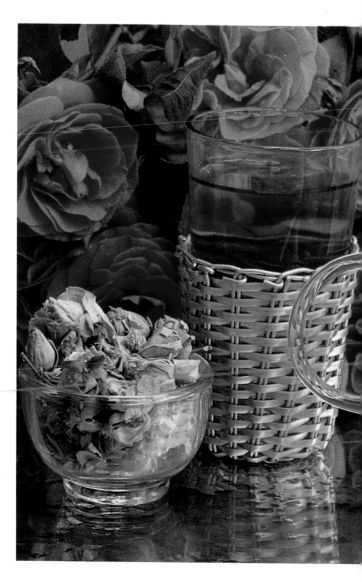

Purple sage tisane

The botanical name for sage – *salvia* – is
derived from the Latin word for healing. This
herb has always been connected with good
health and a long life. It is astringent and
antiseptic. An infusion of sage can be drunk as
a tea or used as a gargle to help a sore throat.
The purple leaves of this herb have a potent
aroma. Alternatively, make a tea using 5ml/1tsp
each of dried or one sprig of fresh sage and
thyme with 250ml/8fl oz/1 cup water.

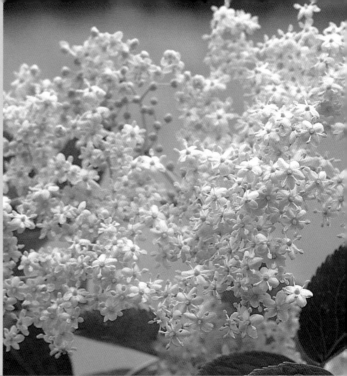

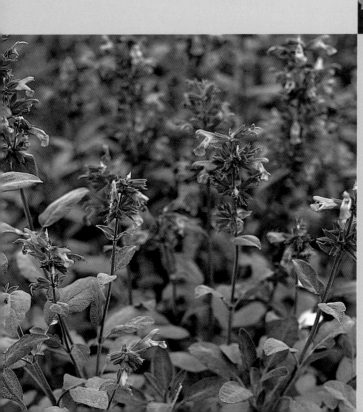

Elderflower, chamomile and peppermint tea

At the onset of a cold, a tea made with these
three herbs will help to relieve feverishness. If
you use dried herbs, you will need 2.5ml/½ tsp
of each per 250ml/8fl oz/1 cup of water. Add a
pinch of lavender for its calming effect, a
sprinkling of ground ginger for its warming
effect, a little honey to sweeten and a slice of
lemon. Peppermint aids digestion, so teas are
best drunk after a meal.

Horehound infusion

This herb has been used as a remedy for chesty coughs and colds since Roman times. The bitter juice extracted from the flowers and leaves is used as a traditional cough medicine ingredient. As well as being made into an infusion for drinking and gargling, it was formerly added to sugar syrup and boiled down to make cough candy. Add the chopped fresh or dried leaves to 250ml/8fl oz/1 cup of boiling water. Sweeten with honey or lemon.

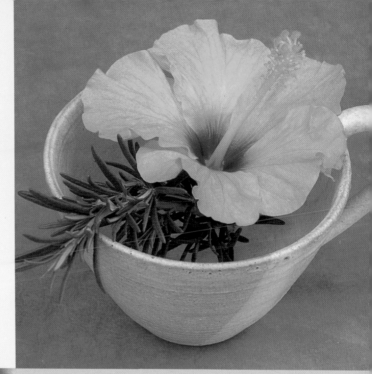

Hibiscus and rose-hip

Like rose-hips, the hibiscus flower is a useful source of vitamin C, so both are valuable in keeping cold viruses at bay. The two can be combined in an infusion. Top, tail and chop two rose-hips, then add them to 5ml/1tsp dried flower petals. Add 250ml/8fl oz/1 cup boiling water and leave to infuse. Note that Hibiscus sino-chinensis is an ornamental flower not suitable for making tea. Hibiscus reduces feverishness and soothes coughs.

Thyme infusion

The strong antiseptic properties of thyme are well established and are good for combating chest infections. Both the leaves and the flowering tops of the stems can be used for infusions. Use 5ml/1 tsp dried thyme, or 10ml/2 tsp fresh, per 250ml/8fl oz/ 1 cup of boiling water. Thyme tea has a warming effect and can be used for stomach chills. It also aids the digestion of fatty foods through the body.

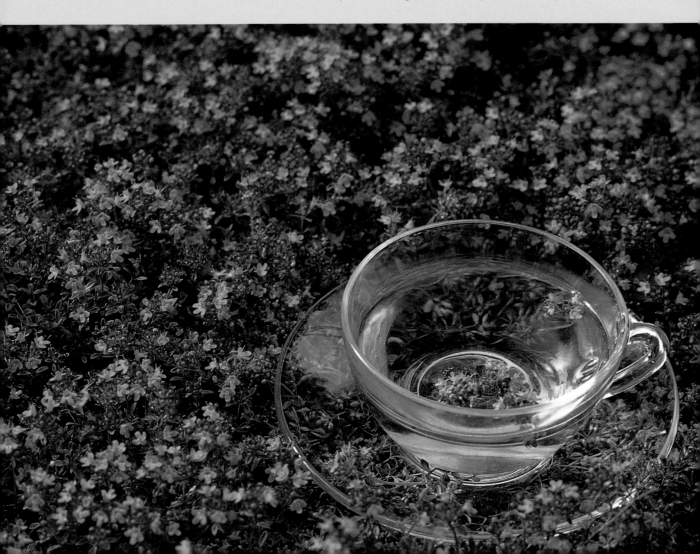

Sage, honey and lemon tea

Honey and lemon are well-known comforters, helping to soothe sore throats and combat coughs. When added to sage tea, they make a comforting traditional treatment for colds, coughs and sore throats. Add 25g/1oz sage leaves to 30ml/2 tbsp clear honey and the juice of a lemon, then dilute with 600ml/ 1 pint/2½ cups boiling water. Cover and leave to infuse for about 20–30 minutes. Strain and drink hot.

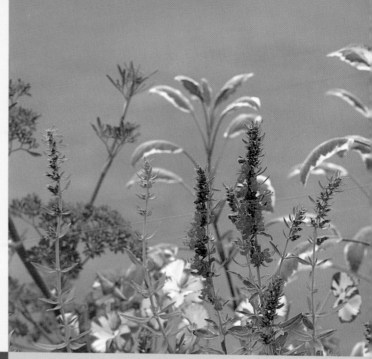

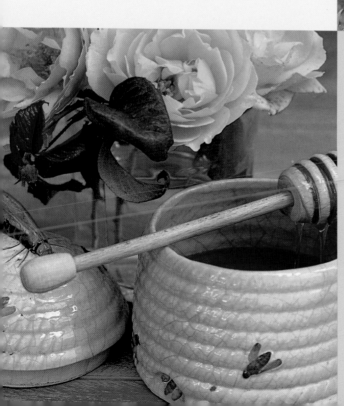

Hyssop tisane

For a cough or sore throat, use a few fresh or 5ml/1 tsp dried leaves and flowers, with 250ml/ 8fl oz/1 cup of boiling water to make an infusion. Hyssop is bitter, so sweeten this tea with honey and add a little freshly squeezed orange juice, which will also provide valuable vitamin C. The fresh flowers, used alone, make a tisane which is a beautiful pale aquamarine colour. Hyssop has expectorant properties, promotes sweating and is anti-catarrhal.

teas for zest and energy

The food we eat provides the energy we need to get us through the day, but frequently we are left without the surplus we would like, and often we feel too exhausted to tackle the ordinary tasks of day-to-day living with any enthusiasm. Eating a diet rich in fruit and vegetables, nuts, seeds, legumes, pulses and carbohydrate will help sustain our physical bodies. Conversely exercise, which we often feel too tired to do, creates more energy, releasing the "feel-good factor" in our bodies and providing a different focus for our attention, even if it is only for a short time. You can help yourself too by cutting down on stimulants, such as caffeine, which tend to exhaust both body and mind. Herbal teas or decoctions can be drunk instead, to support the nervous system and restore energy of all kinds.

Lemon and orange tea

Citrus fruit adds a fresh zestiness to tea and this
blend, with its addition of dried orange and lemon
rind, is ideal for drinking on a summer's afternoon.
For a more pronounced flavour, one or two drops
of orange and lemon essential oils can be added.

Recipe

thinly pared rind of 1 lemon and 1 orange
115g/4oz Ceylon tea leaves

1 Cut the lemon and orange rind into fine ribbons
and allow it to dry slowly in a warm, dry place.
2 Mix the dried rind with the Ceylon tea and
store in an airtight container.
3 Make a cupful of tea as you would for ordinary
tea leaves.

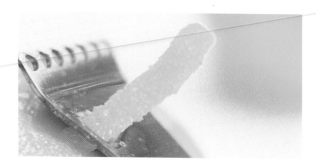

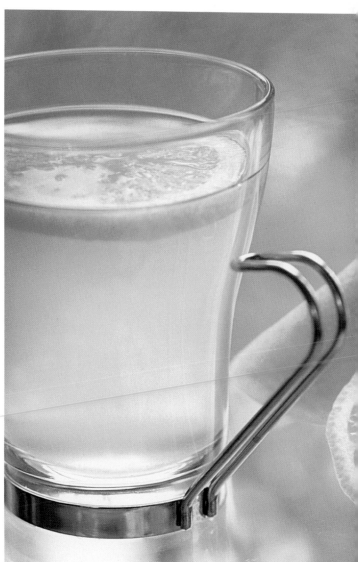

Lemon verbena tea

The essential oil of this plant is used by the perfume industry for its invigorating scent. The fresh or dried leaves of lemon verbena make an uplifting drink with a lively flavour which will help to wake up your system. Add a few fresh leaves, or 5ml/1 tsp dried to a 250ml/8fl oz/1 cup of boiling water. It makes a pale golden, lemony tea which is wonderfully refreshing. Add a little honey for extra flavour and sweetness.

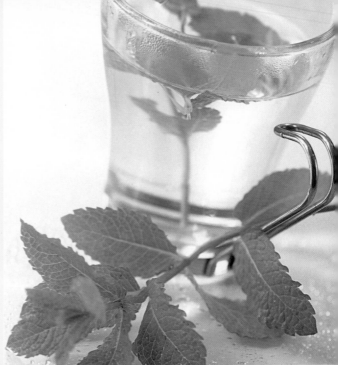

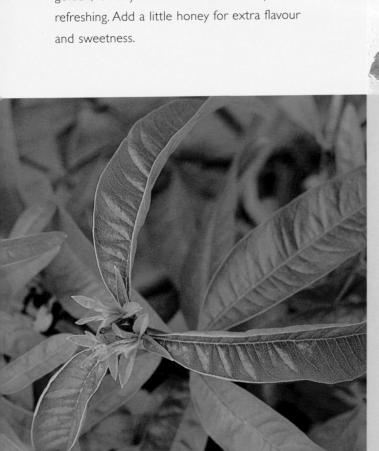

Mint tea

There are 25 species of mint in all, several of which can be used to make distinctive herbal infusions. Peppermint tea is gently stimulating when drunk first thing in the morning. It is also well known as an aid to digestion. Spearmint is the most popular mint for culinary purposes and makes a delicious tea with a zingy, uplifting taste. For the best flavour, use a few freshly picked leaves and add to 250ml/8fl oz/1 cup boiling water. Sweeten with a little honey.

Rosemary tisane

This familiar garden plant contains several active, aromatic oils. It is a sturdy evergreen shrub, and fresh sprigs can be cut all year round. The action of rosemary is stimulating as it increases the supply of blood to the brain, keeping the mind clear and aiding concentration. It will also relax nervous tension and combat fatigue. Add a small sprig to a 250ml/8fl oz/1 cup of boiling water or 10ml/2 tsp of the dried herb. Leave to infuse.

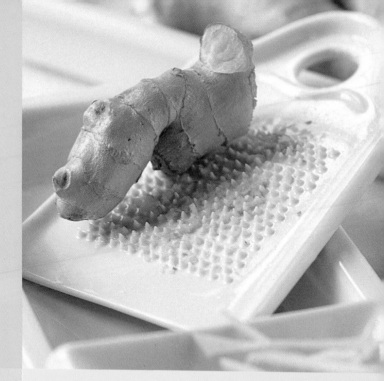

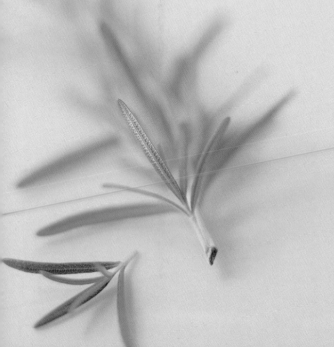

Damiana, ginger and vervain tea

Ginger is one of the oldest and most popular herbal medicines. The root is spicy, peppery and fragrant, making it a warming addition to a cup of tea. Damiana stimulates the nervous and hormonal systems, while vervain releases tension and stress (do not take vervain if you have liver disease). Use 2.5ml/½tsp each dried damiana and vervain and infuse in 250ml/ 8fl oz/1 cup boiling water. Flavour it with a few slices of fresh ginger and drink two cups a day.

teas for calm and sleep

There are many types of insomnia that affect people. If you can't sleep it is best to experiment with various remedies to find the herb, or combination of herbs, that suits you best. If you haven't been sleeping well for a long period, try taking a tonic for your nervous system to improve the long-term situation. Drink teas made from relaxing herbs in the evening. Lavender oil in a hot bath before bed and on your pillow will help, and you could also try a hop pillow. Remember to allow time at the end of the day to relax and wind down.

Chamomile, vervain and lemon balm tisane

Put 5ml/1 tsp each dried chamomile, vervain and lemon balm into a pot and infuse in 600ml/1 pint/2½ cups boiling water. Drink a cup after supper, then warm the rest and drink before going to bed. If you continue to have problems sleeping, add a decoction of 5ml/1 tsp valerian root or 2.5ml/½ tsp dried hops or Californian poppy to the herb blend.

Chamomile and peppermint tea

A perfect bedtime combination, as chamomile is a gentle sedative and peppermint is an excellent aid to digestion. Make a herb blend using 75g/3oz dried chamomile flowers and 25g/1oz dried peppermint leaves, then use 5ml/1 tsp per 250ml/8fl oz/1 cup of boiling water. If you prefer to drink chamomile tea without the addition of peppermint, you could try adding a pinch of lavender, which is also relaxing.

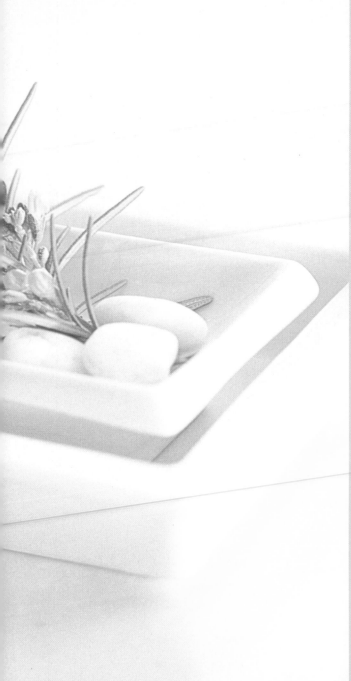

Limeflower and elderflower tea

Soothing limeflower is said to help lower blood pressure, and help relieve anxiety. Limeflower, also known as linden, has always been a popular drink in Europe, especially in France. Combined with delicately flavoured elderflower it makes a pleasant bedtime tea. Blend the dried flowers in equal quantities, then use 5ml/1 tsp per 250ml/8fl oz/1 cup of boiling water. Add a dash of grated nutmeg for flavour, and sweeten to taste with honey.

Valerian infusion

Use the dried and shredded root of white-flowered *Valeriana officinalis* to make a decoction to calm the nerves. Valerian has a powerful sedative effect and reduces the nervous tension and anxiety that hinder sleep. It is also said to lower blood pressure. Using 10ml/2 tsp to a 250ml/8fl oz/1 cup of water, simmer gently for 20 minutes in a covered, non-aluminium pan. Leave to cool then strain. Re-heat and drink just before you go to bed.

teas for headaches, anxiety and depression

Headaches can develop for a number of reasons, and are often a symptom of anxiety or stress; but there are other reasons such as nasal congestion caused by colds, eyestrain, tension, tiredness, poor posture creating tense muscles, too much alcohol, and high blood pressure, to name just a few. Think carefully about the reason you may have a headache before working out how to treat it. If your headache is persistent with no obvious cause, seek medical help. Herbal teas can help alleviate many of the symptoms of headaches and anxiety, and help you deal with depression by lifting the spirits or calming the nerves with their uplifting scents or therapeutic healing qualities.

Lemon balm tea

For lemon balm tea, always use the freshly gathered herb, which is easy to grow in the garden, as the scent, flavour and therapeutic properties are lost when the leaves are dried and stored. Lemon balm has a long tradition as an anti-depressant, and is also helpful for tension headaches and indigestion. It has a gentle sedative effect, so is helpful in calming anxiety.

Recipe

30ml/2 tbsp fresh lemon balm
600ml/1 pint/2½ cups boiling water

1 Put the lemon balm into a pot and pour on the boiling water.

2 Allow to steep for 10 minutes, then strain. Drink one cup three times a day.

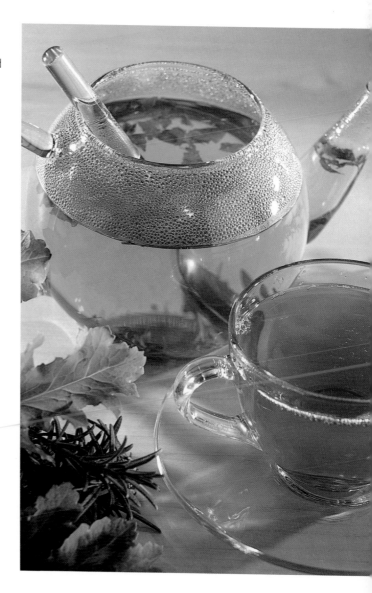

Licorice root tea

When you are anxious or when emotional demands leave you exhausted, a blend of herbs can support your nervous system. Mix equal quantities of oats, licorice root, St John's wort and skullcap. Add a smaller amount of betony. Put 15ml/1 tbsp of this mixture into a pot and add 600ml/1 pint/2½ cups boiling water. Allow to steep for 10 minutes. Drink two cups a day. Do not take this tea if you are pregnant or have high blood pressure.

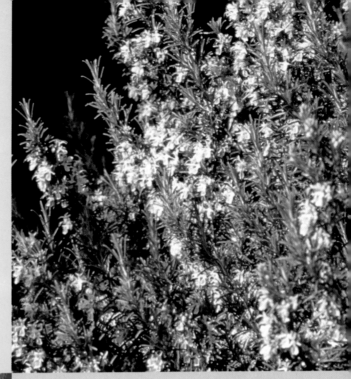

Rosemary and wood betony tisane

Fresh rosemary makes a pleasant tasting tea which is invigorating and refreshing. Rosemary clears the head and eases depression, helping you to deal with difficult times. It improves the circulation and relieves headaches and respiratory problems. Use one or two small sprigs per 250ml/8fl oz/1 cup of boiling water. You can also add a few wood betony leaves to rosemary tea to help relieve nervous tension.

St John's wort tea

Traditionally, St John's wort was considered to be magically protective and a remedy for melancholy. It is now well known for its anti-depressant action. Tea can be made using the flowering tops of the plant, either a few fresh sprigs or 5ml/1 tsp dried with 250ml/8fl oz/ 1 cup of boiling water. It helps to relieve nervous tension and anxiety as well as lifting depression. St John's wort was traditionally gathered on June 23rd to protect against evil.

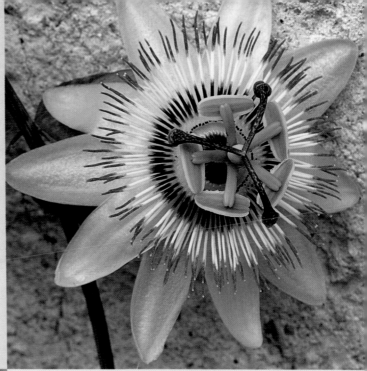

Passionflower tisane

Cut and dried when fruiting, for use in tisanes, passionflower has sedative properties and will relieve nervous conditions such as palpitations, and insomnia. You could also try wood betony vervain, valerian and motherwort. Put 5ml/ 1 tsp of each of two dried herbs that suit you into a pot with 2.5ml/½ tsp passionflower and add 600ml/1 pint/2½ cups boiling water. Leave to steep for 10 minutes. Drink one cup three times a day; continue for two to four weeks.

tonic teas

If you have been ill, it's easy to forget that even if your symptoms have disappeared your body still needs time to recover. Your immune system will be depleted and if you do not give yourself time to recoup what has been lost, you could become vulnerable to recurrent infections. The old-fashioned concept of a tonic is useful for these times. Oats and St John's wort support the nervous system, vervain helps relaxation and digestion, and licorice and borage restore the adrenal glands.

Uplifting tea

This strengthening tea can be flavoured with peppermint or licorice to taste (but avoid licorice if you suffer from high blood pressure).

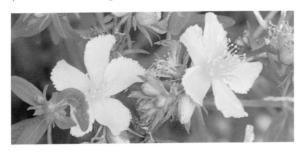

Recipe

2.5ml/½ tsp each dried porridge oats, St John's wort, vervain and a few fresh borage flowers
600ml/1 pint/2½ cups boiling water

1 Put all the herbs into a pot and pour on the water. Leave to steep for 10 minutes, then strain.
2 Drink three or four cups of this blend, warm, each day for at least three weeks.

left St John's Wort is frequently used to treat depression.

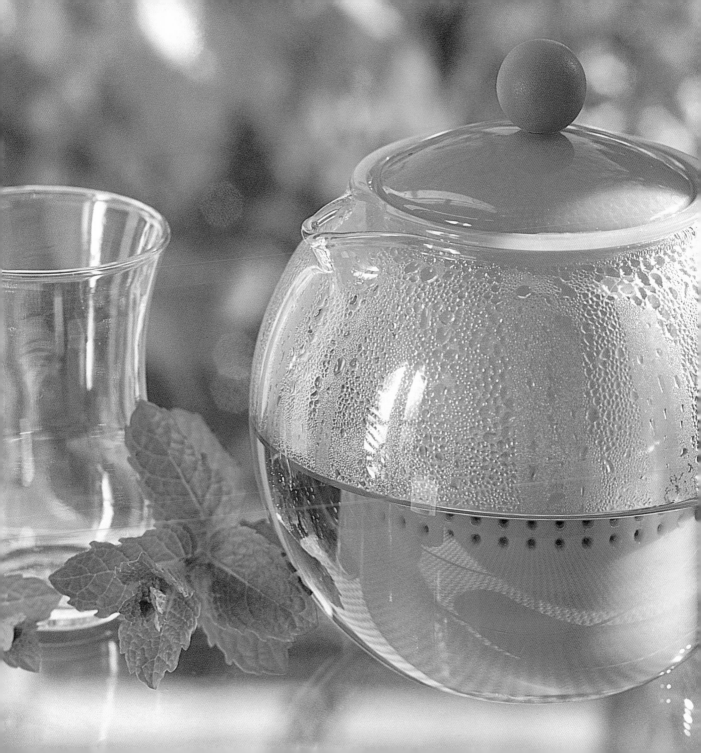

Restorative tea

Make a blend of equal parts dried St John's
wort, porridge oats and damiana. Put 10ml/
2 tsp of the mixture into a pot and add
600ml/1 pint/2½ cups boiling water. Allow to
steep for 10 minutes. Drink a cup of this tea
three times a day. Damiana is harvested when
in flower and is dried for use as an anti-
depressant, to relieve anxiety and to improve
sexual function. It is a helpful tonic for the
nervous system.

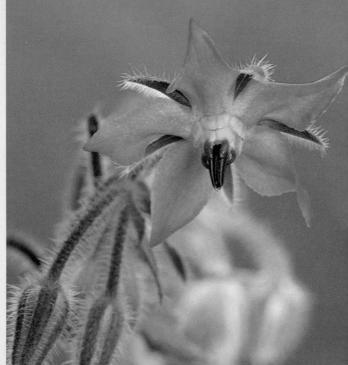

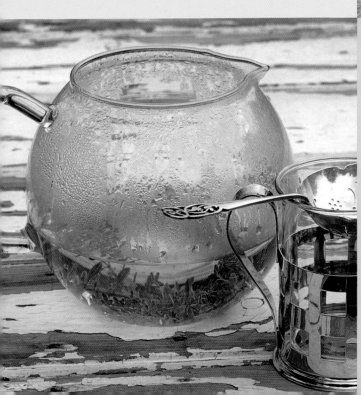

Borage flower tea

However well you cope with what life throws
at you, it's important to remember to look
after yourself when additional demands are
made on you. Traditionally associated with
courage, a drink of borage will raise the spirits
particularly in stressful times. Put 10ml/2 tsp
fresh borage flowers and 2.5ml/½ tsp dried
passionflower into a cup. Add 250ml/8fl oz/
1 cup of boiling water. Sweeten to taste and
drink one cup three times a day.

Soothing tea

Stress can cause many everyday symptoms such as aching muscles from holding yourself in a tense position, tiredness from worrying and tension. To relax the tension and soothe your head, put 2.5ml/½ tsp dried wood betony with the same of dried lavender or rosemary into a cup. Add 250ml/8fl oz/1 cup boiling water and leave for 10 minutes. Strain and drink. Take no more than one or two cups a day. Do not take this tea if you are pregnant.

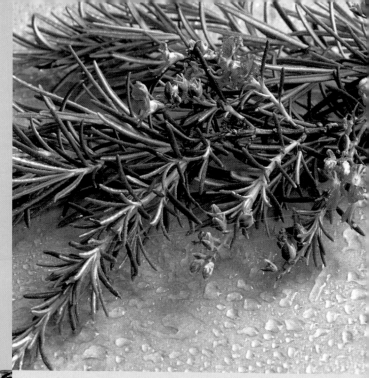

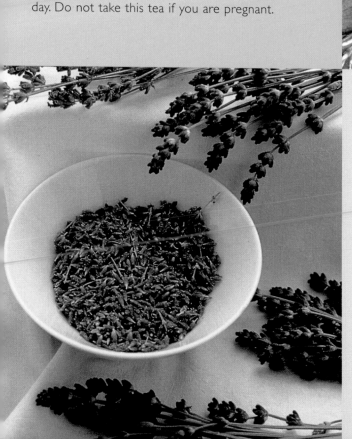

Winter brightener

There is no better herb to take than St John's Wort if you need a tonic for winter blues, when sunlight is in short supply. The addition of rosemary will improve the circulation and keep your mind clear. Combine 10ml/2 tsp dried St John's wort with 5ml/1 tsp dried or 10ml/2 tsp fresh rosemary. Add 250ml/8fl oz/1 cup boiling water and allow to steep for 10 minutes. Drink one cup a day throughout the winter.

Stinging nettle tea

Nettles make a tried and tested tonic tea to cleanse a sluggish system after winter. While an unpopular weed, the stinging nettle has proved to be an important nutritious and medicinal herb. It may also help to alleviate rheumatism and arthritic aches and pains. Chop a handful of young nettle leaves and infuse in 600ml/1 pint/2½ cups boiling water. Allow to steep for 10 minutes then strain. Drink one cup three times a day.

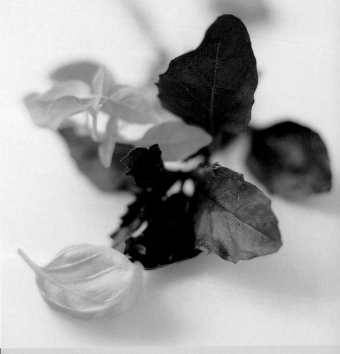

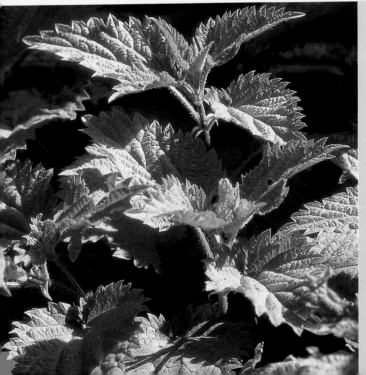

Basil infusion

Calming to the nervous system, basil also helps to relieve nausea and has anti-depressant and antiseptic properties. The leaves do not retain their flavour when dried, so are best used fresh. Add three or four fresh leaves to a 250ml/8fl oz/1 cup of boiling water and steep for 10 minutes. Basil has an overall calming effect, easing sickness and cramps and aiding indigestion. Diluted essential oil makes an effective massage to alleviate depression.

Hangover tea remedy

If you are suffering from a hangover, a bitter herb such as vervain will stimulate the liver and hurry along its detoxification work. It is also important to drink plenty of water and take extra vitamin C. Put 5ml/1 tsp vervain and 2.5ml/½ tsp lavender flowers (which aid digestion) into a pot. Add 600ml/1 pint/2½ cups boiling water. Allow to steep for 10 minutes. Strain and sweeten with a little honey if you wish. Do not drink this tea if you have liver disease.

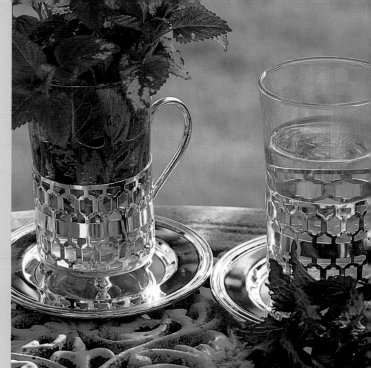

Butterfly blend

If your stomach is in a knot because you are stressed or nervous, ease it with a herbal blend. Put 5ml/1 tsp each dried lemon balm, chamomile flowers and peppermint into a pot and add 600ml/1 pint/2½ cups boiling water. Allow to steep for 10 minutes. Strain and drink up to three times a day or after meals. Hops can be added to settle the stomach, but only in the evening as they have a sedative effect – avoid them if you are depressed.

fruit and flower drinks

While fruit is a nutritious and familiar ingredient in drinks of all kinds, flowers have also long been used to flavour drinks such as cordials, wines, liqueurs and brandy. Cordial waters made of roses, violets, borage and other flowers were recommended as restoratives by the herbalists of the 17th century. Sparkling elderflower and elderflower cordial are perhaps two of the best known floral drinks, but wild flowers such as primrose, cowslip, clary sage, clover, meadowsweet, broom, hawthorn blossom and honeysuckle were all harvested in the past to make wine in season. Dandelions and hops were brewed into both wine and beer, while hops and cowslips were also combined with honey to make mead.

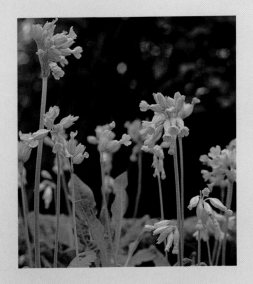

left Cowslips were once used to make floral drinks. Never collect flowers from the wild, always grow your own for home use.

Flower teas or tisanes are light and fragrant refreshing drinks to be enjoyed hot or cold. Lemon can be added for extra flavour and honey can be used to sweeten them. The coloured petals produce drinks of delicate hues such as clear pinks and pale blues.

Many flowers are suitable to make teas with, such as dandelion, rose petal, dill flowers, lemon verbena, lavender, jasmine, peppermint, bergamot and hibiscus. Just take a small quantity of clean flowers (in the case of lemon verbena, peppermint and bergamot you can add a few leaves as well), and add a cup of boiling water. Allow to infuse for about four minutes, then strain to remove the flowers. Drink either warm or chilled.

Bergamot infusion

The Native American Oswegan tribe traditionally made tea from bergamot leaves. After the Boston Tea Party of 1773, American settlers adopted this practice as a substitute for tea. Bergamot flowers have the same flavour as the leaves but they are sweeter and a little more scented. The infusion, known as "Oswego Tea" is taken as a digestive. Use two to three fresh flower heads or 5ml/1 tsp dried flowers to 250ml/8fl oz/1 cup of boiling water.

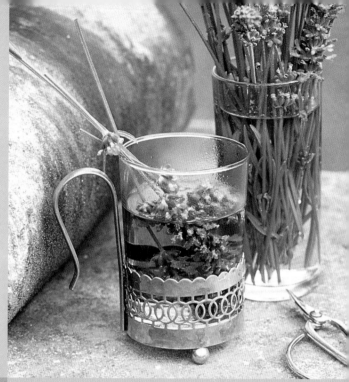

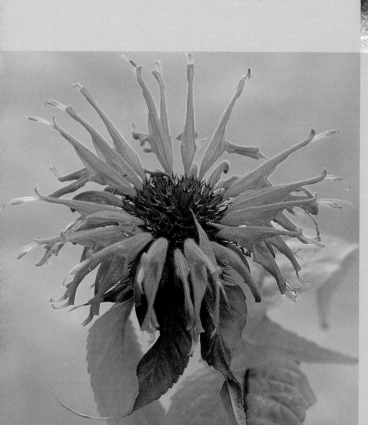

Lavender tisane

Place two or three sprigs of lavender flowers, fresh or dried, in a cup and pour on 250ml/ 8fl oz/1 cup boiling water. Allow to infuse for up to four minutes before removing the flowers. Lavender tea should not be made too strong. It has a beautiful pale blue colour and an uplifting scent which helps relieve anxiety and nervous exhaustion. Take one cup before bedtime as an aid to sleeplessness. Lavender raises the spirits and has relaxing properties.

Hibiscus and rosemary tea

The flowers of the hibiscus have an exotic appeal, with their exquisite colouring and wide papery petals. *Hibiscus sabdariffa*, which is used for tea, is a tender plant that does not grow easily in cold climates. To make hibiscus tea use dried hibiscus and add 5ml/1 tsp to a 250ml/8fl oz/1 cup of boiling water. To enliven the flavour, add a sprig of rosemary. Allow the mix to steep for four minutes, then strain and drink. This infusion can also be drunk chilled.

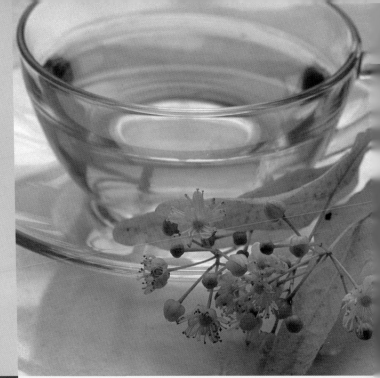

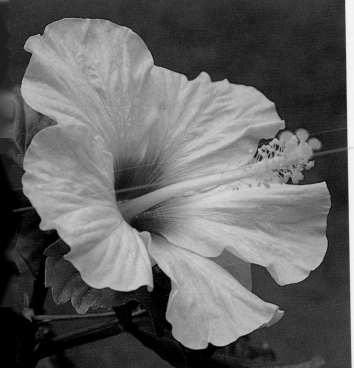

Lime blossom tisane

If you are using fresh lime flowers, pick them as they begin to open. Use five or six fresh flowers for each cup and add 250ml/8 fl oz/ 1 cup hot, but not boiling, water. Steep for no longer than four minutes, then strain. Lime blossom tisane has a delicate pale lemon colour and a creamy taste and can be drunk either hot or chilled, with a slice of lemon. Sweeten with honey. It is helpful for coughs, catarrh and feverishness, and as a digestive.

Rose petal tisane

Cultivated for thousands of years, roses were once valued as much for their medicinal and culinary qualities as for their fragrance. In AD77 the Roman writer Pliny listed over 30 disorders as responding to treatment with preparations of rose. Red rose petals were still being used as ingredients for pharmaceutical preparations until the 1930s.

The petals of scented roses make a delicate infusion that tastes less astringent than rose-hip tea.

Recipe

5ml/1 tsp dried rose petals
600ml/1 pint/2½ cups boiling water

1 Put the rose petals into a pot and pour on the boiling water.

2 Leave to steep for about four minutes, then strain.

Rose petal tea

China tea is a good base tea to which rose petals can be added. Together they make a delicious drink. This tea looks very pretty when poured unstrained into tea glasses, so that the petals and tea leaves are visible at the bottom of the glass.

Recipe

15g/½oz scented dried rose petals
115g/4oz Oolong tea

1 Mix the dried rose petals into the tea and store the blend in an airtight container.

2 Make up a cupful as you would for ordinary tea.

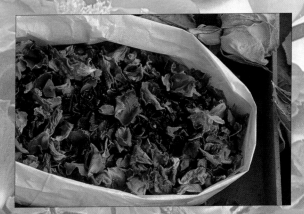

Rose-hip tonic wine

Traditionally, hedgerow rose-hips were gathered to make wine, but if you do not live in the country you could grow a hedge of *Rosa rugosa,* which produces exceptionally large, round hips, if you have a garden.

Recipe

500g/1¼lb/4½ cups rose-hips
2.25 litres/½ gallon/10 cups boiling water
500g/1¼lb/1¼ cups sugar
juice of ½ lemon and ½ orange
7g/¼oz fresh yeast

1 Chop the hips in a food processor and put into a plastic bowl. Pour over the water and stir. Let stand for three days, stirring daily, then strain.
2 Heat the sugar with the lemon and orange juice. Add to the rose-hip juice and pour into a fermenting jar.
3 Cream the yeast with a little liquid, leave to ferment then add to the wine. Add more boiled, cooled water to bring the liquid to 2.5cm/1in from the top of the jar. Fit an airlock and leave in a warm place to ferment. Decant into a clean jar, leave for another three months, then bottle.

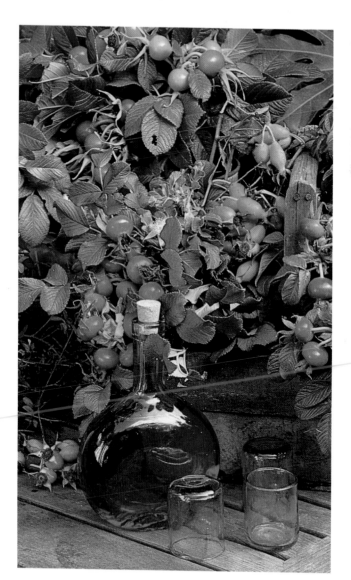

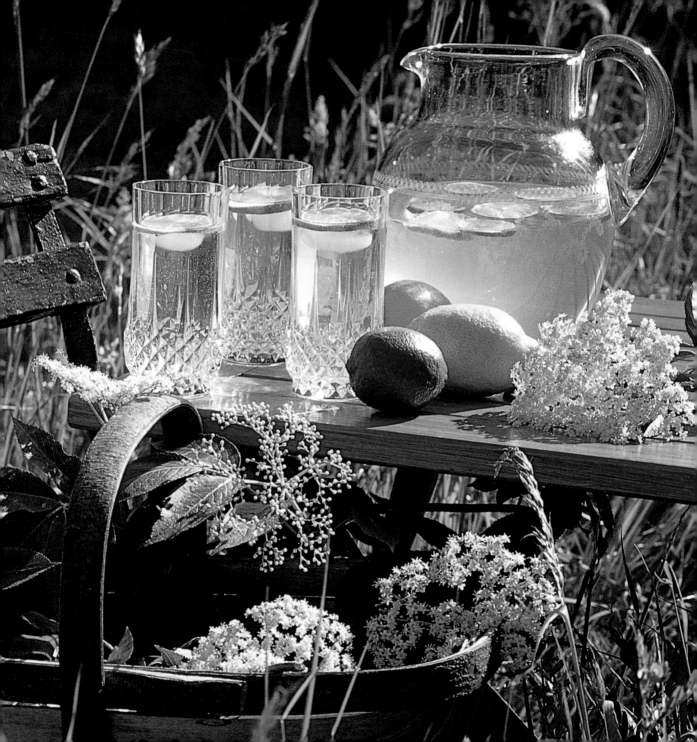

Elderflower cordial

Soothe summer colds with delicious elderflowers. Elderflowers are anti-catarrhal, and limes, are high in vitamin C content.

Recipe
10 fresh elderflower heads
2–3 limes, sliced
675g/1½lb/3 cups sugar
5ml/1 tsp citric acid
5ml/1 tsp cream of tartar
1 litre/1¾ pints/4 cups boiling water

1 Wash and pick over the elderflowers thoroughly. Put them into a large bowl with the sliced limes. Add the sugar, citric acid and cream of tartar. Set aside for two hours.
2 Pour in the boiling water and leave to stand for 24 hours. Strain the syrup into sterilized bottles and cork. The cordial will keep in the refrigerator for two to three months. To serve, dilute with about twice as much chilled still or sparkling water.

right **The flowers of the elder tree have a musk-scent when they appear in early summer.**

Elderflower drink

This delicious, effervescent summer drink has a flavour reminiscent of muscatel wine.

Recipe
4.5 litres/1 gallon/20 cups water
500g/1¼lb sugar
6–8 fresh elderflower heads
2 lemons, sliced
30ml/2 tbsp white wine vinegar

1 Heat half the water to just below boiling point and add the sugar. Stir to dissolve, add the rest of the water and leave to cool. Add the remaining ingredients and leave to stand for 24–48 hours.
2 Strain into strong glass bottles and cork tightly. The drink will be ready to serve in about six days.

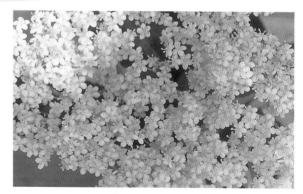

Elderberry rob

Easy to find in the countryside elderberries are rich in vitamins A and C. Take with lemon juice, diluted to taste in hot water, to relieve a feverish cold and support the immune system. Keep refrigerated for several months.

Recipe
1kg / 2¼ lb elderberries
350g / 12oz / 1½ cups sugar
grated rind and juice of 1 orange
10 coriander seeds, crushed
1 cinnamon stick

1 Put all the ingredients into a pan and heat gently until the sugar is dissolved. Simmer for about 20 minutes. Strain and bottle.

Old-fashioned lemonade

Nothing matches fresh, home-made lemonade. Slightly sharp, it makes a most refreshing drink. Lemon balm can be added to enhance the flavour and for the benefit of its relaxing and digestive properties.

Recipe
3 lemons, thinly sliced
675g / 1½ lb / 3½ cups sugar
1.2 litres / 2 pints / 5 cups water
25g / 1oz / ¼ cup citric acid
25g / 1oz / ½ cup fresh lemon balm leaves

1 Put the sliced lemons in a large pan or preserving pan with the sugar and water. Slowly bring to the boil, stirring occasionally until the sugar has dissolved. Boil for 15 minutes then remove from the heat and stir in the citric acid and the lemon balm. Leave to cool.

2 Strain and bottle the lemonade. It can be stored in the refrigerator for up to two weeks. To serve, dilute with twice as much chilled still or sparkling water and add sprigs of fresh lemon balm.

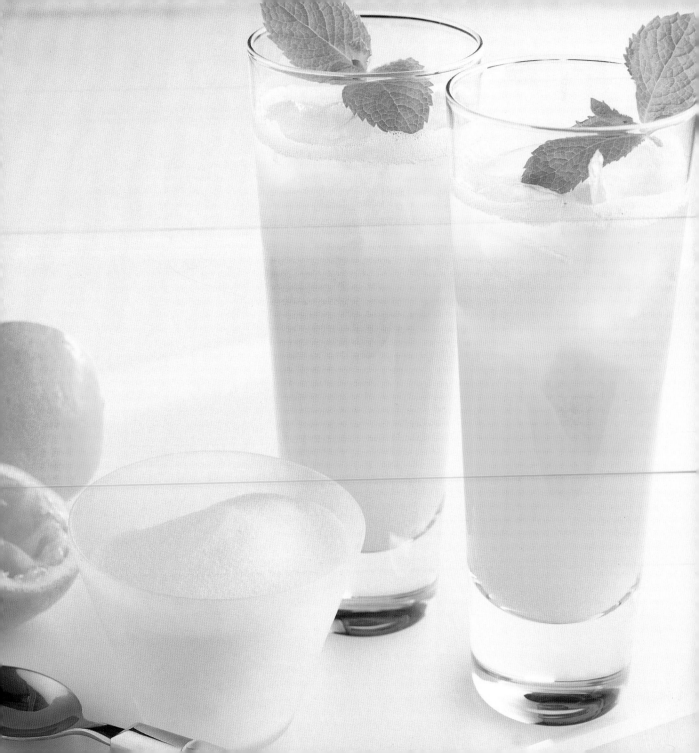

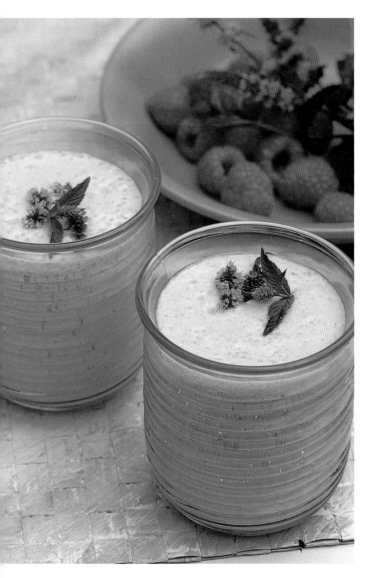

Mint-flower yogurt drink

Raspberries are a rich source of vitamin C. They cleanse the body and remove toxins. Serve this thick, fruity drink chilled. Fresh peaches could be substituted for the raspberries.

Recipe

250ml/8fl oz/1 cup natural yogurt
120ml/4fl oz/½ cup mineral water
75g/3oz raspberries
50g/2oz sugar
4 sprigs flowering mint

1 Place the yogurt, water, fruit and sugar, with two sprigs of mint, in a food processor and purée. Pour into a jug and chill.

2 To serve, pour into two tall glasses and decorate with the remaining sprigs of mint flowers.

Rose petal and strawberry punch

Strawberries are rich in B complex vitamins and vitamin C. They contain potassium and cleanse the skin. Raspberries can be substituted for strawberries if you prefer their flavour.

Recipe

1 bottle rosé wine, chilled
60ml/4 tbsp vodka
75g/3oz strawberries, sliced
handful of fresh, scented rose petals, with the white
    heels at the base removed
1 bottle sparkling mineral water, chilled

1 Pour the wine into a glass punch bowl. Add the vodka and sliced strawberries.
2 Scatter the rose petals over the bowl and chill for an hour. Add the sparkling water before serving.

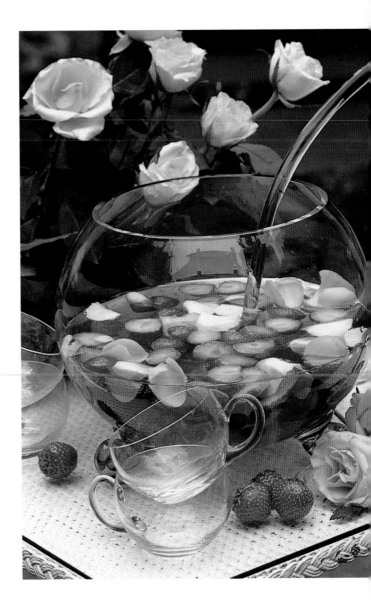

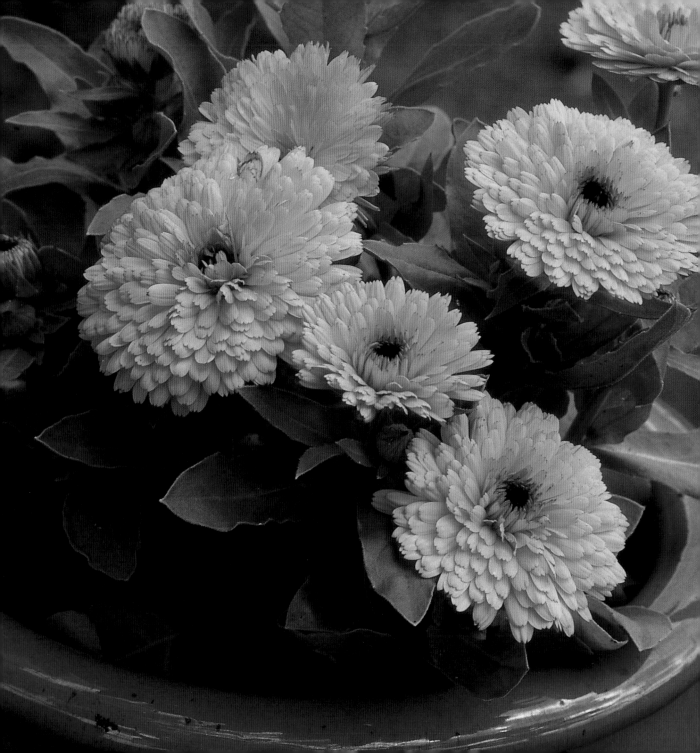

a potted tea garden

If you use a range of herbs specifically to make herbal teas that you find effective, it's useful to be able to pick them fresh in season, and to ensure a good supply of leaves for drying. Herbs are a good addition to any garden, since they can be used for cooking and medicinal purposes as well as for making herbal teas. Many have beautiful foliage and attractive flowers as well as delicious aromas. But if you are growing herbs specifically for herbal teas, grow each herb in its own pot.

Herbs for teas

Although herbs will thrive in most locations, if you have never grown herbs before, just choose a few and purchase small plants from a reputable garden centre, then pot them up into larger containers at home. Dill, borage, caraway and many other herbs are easy to grow from seed. Annual herbs will need to be planted fresh each year. For fully grown plants, use containers with a minimum diameter of 23cm/9in.

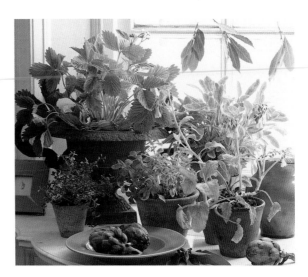

useful herbs to gather

The herbs that follow are particularly useful for common problems. All are hardy, except basil and lemon verbena which need winter protection.

Herbal remedies do not usually work instantly, so give them time to take effect. Seek the advice of a qualified practitioner if symptoms persist.

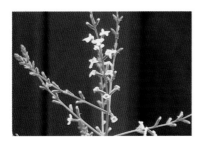

Aloysia triphylla – Lemon verbena

A half-hardy deciduous shrub with rough-textured, strongly lemon-scented, spear-shaped leaves, dotted on the underside with oil glands, which appear in late spring. Racemes of tiny mauve-white flowers appear in late summer. It can grow to 4.5m/15ft. It will survive −5°C/23°F, if it is grown in a sheltered, south-facing site in well-drained soil. Lemon verbena makes a refreshing tea when mixed with other herbs.

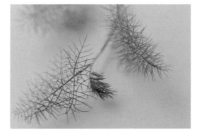

Anethum graveolens – Dill

An aromatic annual, 1m/3ft tall, with a single stem and feathery leaves. It produces terminal umbels of tiny yellow flowers in midsummer and elliptic, flattened seeds. It should not be grown near fennel.

Dill is a cooling, soothing herb. It aids digestion, and prevents constipation. Poultices of the leaves are applied to boils and to reduce swelling and joint pains. Seeds are chewed to cure bad breath.

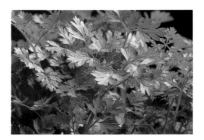

Anthriscus cerefolium – Chervil

A hardy annual, 30–60cm/1–2ft tall, with bright green, finely divided feathery leaves and flat umbels of small white flowers in early summer. It is widely cultivated in warm and temperate climates. It prefers light, moist soil and a sunny situation. Sow seed successionally for a continuous supply.

The leaves of chervil are used to make a mild digestive tea. Its use is mainly culinary.

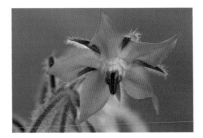

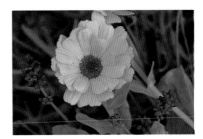

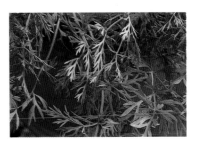

Borago officinalis – **Borage**

A short-lived hardy annual, 60–90cm/ 2–3ft tall, with a sprawling habit. It has hollow, hairy stems, downy leaves and blue star-shaped flowers with black centres. It is attractive to bees. Borage seeds contain gamma-linoleic acid. This important herb is grown as a commercial crop for the oil which is extracted from the seeds. It grows in any soil and prefers a sunny position. It is easy to propagate from seed in spring or autumn, and also self-seeds.

This cooling, anti-inflammatory herb has diuretic properties, and is said to be mildly antidepressant. Used externally, it soothes inflamed skin and is used for mouthwashes and gargles.

Calendula officinalis – **Marigold**

A low-growing annual – to 50cm/20in – with hairy, slightly sticky mid-green leaves and large orange-yellow daisy-like flowers produced throughout summer. Pot marigolds are propagated from seed sown in spring or autumn and are easy to grow. Regular dead-heading ensures a good supply of flowers over a long period. The petals can be used fresh or dried. Marigolds of the Tagetes genus are not related to the pot marigold; many are toxic and should not be used for the same purposes as *Calendula*.

Calendula has antiseptic, anti-inflammatory properties and is antibacterial and antifungal. It adds a refreshing zip to tea.

Carum carvi – **Caraway**

A biennial plant 45–60cm/18–24in tall, caraway has feathery leaves and umbels of white flowers which appear in its second year, followed by ridged seeds. They are a popular culinary flavouring, used in bread, cakes, savoury dishes and pickles. The young leaves can be added to salads. The plant prefers well-drained soil and sun, and is propagated by seed sown in spring, preferably where it is to grow as it does not transplant well.

Caraway seeds are used in infusions and decoctions to treat digestive disorders and to relieve flatulence. If the seeds are chewed they will sweeten the breath.

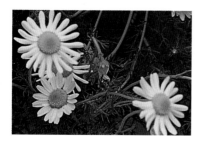

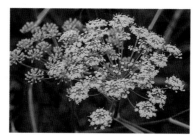

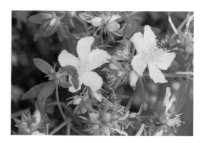

Chamaemelum nobile – Chamomile

An evergreen perennial with finely divided, feathery leaves growing to 15cm/6in. The flowers are borne singly on long stems rising to 30cm/12in. It has an apple-like fragrance, particularly after rain, or when crushed. It prefers light, sandy soil and a sunny position. Chamomile can be grown from seed, but the usual method is by division of runners or "offsets".

Chamomile has anti-inflammatory properties and is soothing and sedative. As a tea it eases nausea and indigestion and promotes sound sleep. Chamomile tea may help painful menstruation. An infusion washed through fair hair will give added shine too!

Foeniculum vulgare – Fennel

A graceful, aromatic perennial, up to 2m/6ft tall, with erect, hollow stems and mid-green, feathery foliage: the leaves are pinnate with threadlike leaflets. Umbels of yellow flowers are borne in summer, followed by ovoid, ridged, yellow-green seeds. The whole plant is strongly scented with aniseed. Fennel likes a sandy soil in full sun. It does not always survive very cold or wet winters. Propagate from seed sown in spring. It should not be grown near dill, as the two plants will cross-pollinate.

Fennel tea aids digestion, and is said to increase the production of breast milk in nursing mothers. It will soothe gum disorders and sore throats.

Hypericum perforatum – St John's wort

A hardy perennial, about 30–60cm/1–2ft tall. The stems are erect, woody at the base, with small linear-oval leaves and yellow flowers. The plant grows in well-drained, dryish soil in full sun or partial shade. Propagation by division is the easiest method, but it can also be grown from seed.

The flowers are used fresh or dried. St John's Wort is an anti-depressant, said to have calming qualities. Teas are taken for anxiety and nervous tension. It has antiseptic and anti-inflammatory properties.

St John's Wort is known to affect some medications, so be careful to always check with your doctor before using it in conjuction with prescribed medicines.

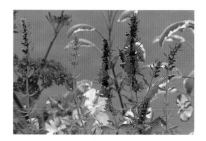

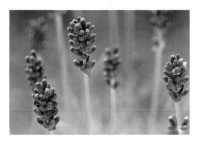

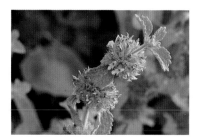

Hyssopus officinalis – Hyssop

Classed as a semi-evergreen because it loses some foliage in severe winters, hyssop is a bushy perennial, about 60–90cm/2–3ft tall. The stems are woody at the base with small, dark green, linear leaves and dense spikes of deep blue flowers in late summer, which are very attractive to bees. There are also forms with pink and white flowers. It likes to grow in well-drained to dry soil in a sunny position. Propagate by seed sown in spring or by cuttings taken in summer. Prune back hard in spring to prevent it becoming straggly.

Infusions of hyssop are good for colds, coughs and chest infections. It has expectorant properties, and is anti-catarrhal and antibacterial.

Lavandula spp. – Lavender

This shrub has been in cultivation for so long that accurate identification of species is not always easy, and most of the plants grown in gardens are hybrids or cultivars. *L. angustifolia*, common lavender, has small purple flowers, grows to 60–90cm/2–3ft, and is effective for medicinal purposes. It has many attractive cultivars, which are more fragrant and decorative. Lavender requires well-drained soil and full sun.

Lavender has calming and soothing properties. It will ease a headache and can alleviate the symptoms of anxiety and nervous exhaustion. Its uplifting scent makes this a pleasant, sweet-tasting drink.

Marrubium vulgare – Horehound

A hardy perennial growing to 60cm/2ft, with erect, branching stems and greeny-grey, soft, downy, toothed leaves. Whorls of small, white tubular flowers appear in the leaf axils in summer. The plant will grow in any soil and prefers a sunny situation. It can be propagated from seed sown in spring, but can be slow to germinate. Alternatively, the roots can be divided in spring. Use the flowering stems fresh or dried.

The bitter juice of horehound has been used as a cough remedy for centuries. Taken as an infusion it will help relieve coughs, colds and chest infections. Combine it with ginger for a warming tea to effectively relieve a cold.

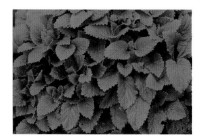

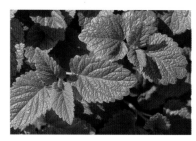

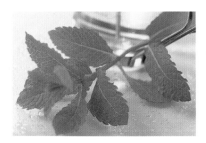

Melissa officinalis – **Lemon balm**

A vigorous, bushy perennial 30–80cm/12–32in tall. Bunches of the plant were once put into empty hives to attract swarms of bees. It has strongly lemon-scented, rough-textured, oval leaves. Inconspicuous clusters of pale yellow flowers appear in the leaf axils in late summer. It will grow in any soil, in sun or partial shade, and it spreads and self-seeds freely. The leaves are best used fresh.

Lemon balm has sedative, relaxing, digestive properties. Tea is taken for nervous anxiety, depression, tension headaches and indigestion. The infusions can be used externally to treat skin irritations, insect bites and stings.

Mentha x piperita – **Peppermint**

A vigorous hardy perennial that grows 30–90cm/1–3ft tall, peppermint has dark green, toothed leaves and whorls of pale pink flowers in summer. It is rich in menthol, which makes it too dominant for general cookery. Peppermint grows in rich, damp soil and partial shade. It is easily propagated by division or by taking root cuttings.

Peppermint tea is a good decongestant and can be used to effectively treat colds.

Peppermint tea should not be taken by pregnant women or by children under the age of ten, unless under professional advice from a qualified herbalist.

Mentha spicata – **Spearmint**

This popular culinary mint grows 30–90cm/1–3ft tall and has brightly coloured green, wrinkled, finely toothed leaves, with a fresh, uncomplicated, not too overpowering mint scent. White or pale mauve flowers are borne in terminal spikes in mid- to late summer. It has been used to flavour food since Roman times. Spearmint grows best in rich, damp soil and partial shade. It is easily propagated by division or by taking root cuttings from early spring and throughout the growing season.

Like peppermint tea, spearmint can be taken as a digestive after a meal. It has a less pungent flavour and is a non-irritant.

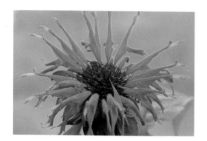

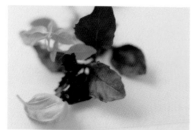

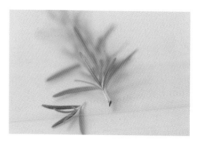

Monarda didyma – **Bergamot**

An aromatic, hardy perennial, 40–90cm/16in–3ft in height, bergamot has soft, downy, greyish-green, oval leaves with serrated edges, and red or mauve flowers in solitary terminal whorls in late summer. It needs humus-rich, damp soil and prefers partial shade, though it will tolerate full sun if it is kept moist. Propagate by division or by seed sown in spring.

The fresh and dried leaves and flowers of the bergamot plant are used to make herbal teas. Bergamot is taken as a digestive tea, and when added to oriental tea leaves will give an "Earl Grey" flavour to the drink. It has a refreshing, uplifting scent.

Ocimum basilicum – **Basil**

A half-hardy annual growing to 20–60cm/8–24in tall, with soft, ovate, bright green leaves. Whorls of small white flowers are borne in terminal racemes in mid- to late summer. Basil is variable and its pungency and flavour vary depending on soil, climate and growing conditions. It requires well-drained, moist, soil and full sun. Propagate from seed. In colder regions it may need to be grown under glass, but flourishes in pots and should be put outside in hot spells for the best flavour.

The leaves of this pungent herb are used to make teas with anti-depressant, soothing and antiseptic properties. Take an infusion to treat a cold.

Rosmarinus officinalis – **Rosemary**

An evergreen shrub which grows to 2m/6ft tall, rosemary has woody branches and strongly aromatic, needle-like foliage. A dense covering of small, tubular, two-lipped flowers appears in spring. Rosemary is a Mediterranean native and thrives on sharply drained, stony soils, requiring little moisture. Although it is frost-hardy it needs a sunny, sheltered position and protection in severe winters. It is easily propagated from semi-ripe cuttings taken in summer. It should be pruned hard in summer.

Rosemary is a restorative, tonic herb with antiseptic, and anti-bacterial properties. It is taken as an infusion to relieve colds, influenza, fatigue and headaches.

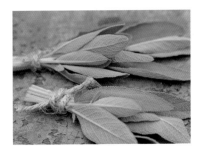

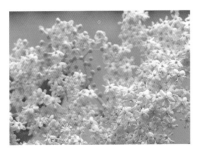

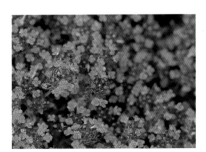

Salvia officinalis – Sage

An evergreen, highly aromatic shrubby perennial, growing to 60cm/2ft tall. It has downy, rough-textured, grey-green, ovate leaves and spikes of tubular, violet-blue flowers in early summer. It needs light, well-drained soil in full sun. It will not always withstand prolonged cold below −10°C/14°F.

It may be propagated from seed. Prune sage in the spring or just after flowering to keep it in good shape. Sage has astringent, antiseptic qualities making it a good infusion to take for sore throats, mouth ulcers, gum disease and as a general tonic.

Sage should not be taken internally by pregnant women.

Sambucus nigra – Elder

A small deciduous tree, growing up to 10m/33ft tall, elder has dull green, pinnate leaves divided into five leaflets. Flat umbels of creamy, musk-scented flowers appear in early summer and are followed by pendulous clusters of spherical black fruits on red stalks in early autumn. The tree can be grown from seed and often self-seeds prolifically. Some ornamental cultivars make attractive garden plants, but these have no medicinal or culinary value.

Elder teas, made from the flowers, are taken for colds, sinusitis, influenza and fevers. The berries are made into syrups which are also taken for colds.

Thymus spp. – Thyme

There are 350 species of thyme, with many hybrids and cultivars. For medicinal purposes, *Thymus vulgaris* (common thyme) and *T. serpyllum* (wild thyme) are the most useful. Common thyme, native to the Mediterranean and southern Europe, is a sub-shrub that grows 30–45cm/12–18in tall with woody stems, small dark green leaves and white or mauve flowers. It can be propagated by seed in spring or cuttings in summer. Thyme needs free-draining, gritty soil and full sun.

Infusions are taken for coughs, colds, chest infections and digestive upsets. Thyme is strongly antiseptic, and antibacterial.

herbs and their uses

Herbal tea	Use
Anise hyssop	The leaves are used to make an infusion to alleviate coughs, colds and indigestion.
Bergamot	A digestive tea.
Calamint	The leaves and flowers are made into an infusion to treat indigestion.
Caraway	The seeds are taken as an infusion to treat digestive disorders and to relieve flatulence.
Chamomile	The flowers are taken as a tea for nausea, indigestion and insomnia. It may help to relieve painful menstruation.
Dill	A cooling, soothing herb that aids digestion and prevents constipation.
Fennel	An infusion of the seeds soothes the digestive system, and is said to increase the production of breast milk in nursing mothers, as well as being settling for the baby.
Fenugreek	Decoctions of the seeds are used for stomach upsets and to ease menstrual pain.
Ginseng	The combined action of its many constituents has a general tonic effect on the whole body.
Hops	Taken as an infusion the dried flowers have sedative and antibacterial properties which help relieve insomnia, nervous tension and anxiety.
Hyssop	Infusions are taken for coughs, colds and chest infections.
Lemon balm	Infusions are taken for nervous anxiety, depression, tension headaches and indigestion.
Lemon verbena	Use the leaves to make a refreshing cup of tea.
Lovage	Use for digestive disorders, colic, flatulence, cystitis and kidney stones.
Meadowsweet	A traditional remedy taken as an infusion, for heartburn, excess acidity and gastric ulcers.
Passionflower	Infusions of the leaves are taken to relieve nervous anxiety and stress.
Peppermint	Peppermint is taken as a tea for colds and to aid digestion,
Rosemary	A restorative tonic herb with antiseptic and antibacterial properties.
Safflower	Tea, infused from fresh or dry flowers is taken to induce perspiration and reduce fevers.
Sage	Infusions are taken as tonics, as an aid to digestion and for menopausal problems.
St John's wort	Infusions are taken for anxiety and nervous tension. St John's wort has antiseptic and anti-inflammatory properties and promotes healing.
Thyme	Infusions are taken for coughs, colds, chest infections and digestive upsets.
Valerian	Taken as a tea, it helps relieve insomnia, nervous tension, anxiety, headaches and indigestion. It is said to lower blood pressure.
Yarrow	Increases perspiration, helps relieve colds and feverish conditions.

index

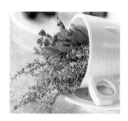